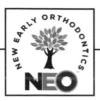

The NEO Way is revolutionizing orthodontics. It represents the most radical change ever in treating children's poor bites and crooked teeth. Traditional orthodontists may have parents wait until teeth and jaws approach full development at around age 11 or 12 before beginning extensive orthodontic braces, which then may require tooth extractions or even surgery.

With New Early Orthodontics, NEO sees children as young as age four, while most facial growth is still ahead, to naturally straighten teeth and form beautiful smiles. Along with habit correction exercises, NEO uses gentle oral appliances worn for only an hour plus sleep time to create straight teeth in the most natural way, eliminating or lessening the need for braces later. The NEO Way is an integrative medical approach and truly is the future of orthodontics!

What happy patients are saying about The NEO Way:

"We love NEO! The whole staff is super friendly and welcoming. Our son has been going here for about a year now. They praise and encourage my son's growth and progress every time we're in."

Tarrah W., Castle Rock, CO

"I highly recommend this revolutionary concept! I wish more orthodontists would get on board with this."

Jennifer P., Parker, CO

"They are super friendly and knowledgeable. Answered all my questions. Love them! Great facility too. And it's working on my daughter's teeth and jaw! Love the holistic approach."

Lindsey S., Highlands Ranch, CO

"We have a nine-year-old son whose front teeth were at a 90-degree angle. Within 6 months of treatment at NEO the results were beyond what we thought possible. We are now 11 months into the treatment and his top and bottom teeth are perfectly aligned. The results are amazing, and we highly recommend NEO."

Mark R., Lutz, FL

"This is such a great place. Staff is amazing. What they can do with kids and the permanent correction of teeth without pulling teeth and minimal to no braces is amazing. Check them out!"

Jeremy R., Parker, CO

"Ever since I've been here my teeth have been improving like crazy! I feel very secure about my smile and my teeth."

Bryce L., Parker, CO

"What an amazing concept this orthodontist has brought to Denver! My daughter's teeth are straightening without braces. I am so impressed and so was my dentist with the progress my daughter has made by wearing her Myobrace. The staff is so friendly and great."

Gabriella B., Aurora, CO

"We went in skeptical if they could really help my kids with their orthodontic problems and they blew us away! They were super friendly and personable and very kid-friendly. After seeing a myofacial therapist for my daughter the previous year, I understand just how important a part the palate and facial muscles can play in the shape and health of your child's mouth. I'm so thankful I found NEO and didn't go the normal 'braces' route. I'm very excited to see the progress my children make with the Myobrace!"

Lydia B., Highlands Ranch, CO

"My twins are both in a NEOBrace and I had braces as a child. I recall many unscheduled, last-minute runs to the orthodontist for wires causing pain. I remember not being able to eat my favorite foods for fear of broken brackets. With the NEOBrace, there are no unscheduled emergency issues and my children can eat what they want without fear of breaking their braces. The extra hour of silence during the day while they wear their NEOBrace is an added benefit to my sanity! Can't recommend NEOBrace enough."

Chris W., Littleton, CO

"I have three kids in the Myobrace appliance. All three were finger or thumb suckers with narrow palates. For my oldest (12), her smile is amazing. Her bite is near perfect. Her dentist even asked if she had braces. She has only been in the Myobrace for about a year. My middle daughter (10) has the narrowest palate and the Myobrace has done wonderful things, but her palate is still too narrow for all her teeth, so in their commitment to providing optimal care, they fit her for an alternative expander. My son has had beautiful expansion with the Myobrace and has made room for his permanent teeth. The service at NEO is amazing. My kids enjoy going and I have recommended them to friends and will continue to do so."

Tiffanie M., Denver, CO

"My 10-year-old daughter has been using the Myobrace for about 7 months. I am amazed at the results. I was told we would have to have teeth pulled and have years of braces. I have another daughter and we have been through this before. It is very expensive and painful for the child. So being a single parent, I am so excited to see how straight her teeth already are! She will most likely never have to go through having teeth pulled, and will likely not wear braces. I have told all her friends and parents and urged them to go to NEO!"

Cherie B., Bennett, CO

"My 7-year-old daughter has been using a Myobrace through NEO for 6 months and we are amazed at the results we've seen with her! Her teeth are coming in straight and she's breathing and sleeping better at night. The staff is incredibly friendly and helpful. My daughter loves NEO and loves her Myobrace. (Can you say that about traditional braces?) She's excited to see how well she's doing at her appointments and she loves the reward points she gets for wearing her Myobrace. We highly recommend NEO and their staff and will have our other children go through treatment there as well."

Hannah F., Highlands Ranch, CO

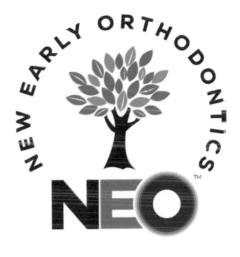

The NEO Way

NEW EARLY ORTHODONTICS

A BETTER WAY TO A MORE
NATURALLY BEAUTIFUL FACE

S. KENT LAUSON, DDS, MS, ORTHODONTIST

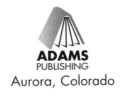

ADAMS
PUBLISHING
Aurora, Colorado

Adams Publishing, LLC
14991 E. Hampden Ave. Suite 300
Aurora, Colorado 80016

First Edition

Publisher's Cataloguing-in-Publication available upon request
Hardcover ISBN: 978-0-9839620-3-8
Ebook ISBN: 978-0-9839620-4-5

Photo credits: Bri Rodriquez, Dakota Patten and Sharon Gilmore

Illustrations: Todd Gilmore

Treatment Credits: All cases shown in NEO Case Studies are patients treated by Dr. Kent Lauson, Dr. Holly Baller and Nichole Griek, Director of Myofunctional Therapy

All cases shown in The Lauson System have been treated by Dr. Kent Lauson and staff at Aurora Orthodontics & TMJ

Cover and Book Design: Patricia Bacall

Editor: Trish Westin

Printed in the United States of America on acid-free paper.

DISCLAIMER

I have attempted to be accurate and thorough in my explanations at every level, and I (along with anyone involved with the publication, distribution, or sale of this book) assume no responsibility. Although there are many statements in this book that show the difference of the treatment we recommend to that of 'traditional' orthodontics, in no way do I insinuate that orthodontists as a group knowingly act to the detriment of their patients. Unfortunately, they do what they have been taught, so if there is a culpability, it lies on the doorsteps of the university specialty training programs who, as a group, have grossly fallen behind the times. **The names in this book have been changed to protect the privacy of the individuals.**

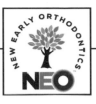

TABLE OF CONTENTS

PART II A: NEO CASE STUDIES, AGES FOUR TO TWELVE 31

PART II B: THE LAUSON SYSTEM CASES
AGES THIRTEEN TO EIGHTEEN   51

PART III: THE LAUSON SYSTEM:
TEN KEYS TO FACIAL HARMONY   61

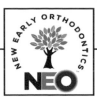

INTRODUCTION

Are you the proud parent of a young child? Do you want to believe your child will have an amazing future with the possibility of realizing many hopes and dreams? If so, then this book is for you. Raising a child can be one of the most challenging endeavors a parent will ever experience. As a parent, you have the awesome opportunity to guide your child in an uncertain world, helping him or her to create a happy and successful life. Along the way, you'll face countless choices that will influence his or her development.

Some of these choices you make for your child will require a financial investment. These can be anything from dance or singing classes to braces. Wait—braces? For your young child? Yes it seems that for most young children braces will be in their future. In fact, studies have shown that as many as 80 percent of all American children will need orthodontic treatment as they gain their final, permanent teeth. This fact alone strikes fear into the hearts of many parents. If this is you, don't despair.

An investment in your child's smile, although somewhat costly, can be one of the most rewarding investments you can make for your child's future. You may think there is little you can do to avoid this expense. You also may ask, "Has orthodontics changed since I was a teenager?" The bad news is that much of the orthodontic profession has changed very little. Many orthodontists are still doing things the way they have been done for decades and using just braces to straighten the teeth. Because a child's mouth keeps developing until adolescence, many parents postpone braces until that time. We call this old-school way of practice "traditional orthodontics."

You may have taken your child to your family dentist and he or she told you to save your money because your child will need braces in the future.

You may have asked, "Isn't there something we can do now?" You have noticed the problem of crooked teeth developing for several years, but your dentist assures you that the orthodontist doesn't even want to see the child until all the permanent teeth are coming in at around age eleven or twelve. This part of orthodontics has been stuck in tradition for many decades.

The truth is that waiting for braces is not the only or best solution. As it turns out, a great deal of progress has been made in the field of orthodontics—so much, in fact, that it is now possible to treat children much earlier. In this way, the child's mouth can develop more naturally, and adult teeth grow in straighter, often without the later need for braces. What a vast improvement this is!

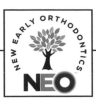

PART I: THE NEO WAY

Have you ever seen something so profound and obvious that you proclaimed, "This makes perfect sense! Why haven't I heard about this before?" Of course, you have! When you see for yourself how NEO is so radically different and better, you'll be compelled to make this bold statement. Welcome to the world of NEO! NEO is an acronym for New Early Orthodontics. The letters NEO also imply something new and something better than the old way of doing things. NEO is revolutionizing orthodontics. It is significantly changing the entire process. It represents the most radical change ever in treating crooked teeth. It is the future of orthodontics and it is available now!

THE NEO WAY will show you how current advances can not only create that coveted "star smile," but even more importantly, how they can make a significant difference in helping your child have a healthier life long after the orthodontist has finished their work. NEO produces the desired result and does so in a more natural way, a way that takes advantage of a child's natural growth and facial development. When all is said and done, this method creates lifetime dental stability—a feat not as likely with the traditional orthodontic approach which often requires wearing retainers for the rest of a person's life.

TRADITIONAL ORTHODONTICS

As it turns out, this old-school orthodontic approach of "wait till age eleven or twelve to do any significant treatment" might be sowing the seeds for future trouble. The traditional "wait and see" approach will likely result in less-desirable treatment options, including extractions and/or surgery, which can be harmful to a child's present and future health. And yet, the old way of treatment, primarily with braces, continues to be the most dominant type of treatment in America.

Just what is this old-school type of treatment? As orthodontists, we went through at least two years of specialty training beyond dental school. We were taught many things, and while most were true, some of the things we were taught do not serve our patients' best interests. The idea that we should wait to treat until all the permanent teeth have come into the mouth is one of those outmoded ideas.

So what is wrong with this approach? Plenty can be wrong with "wait and see" treatment. It starts with the timing of treatment. As much as 90 percent of a child's facial growth has already occurred by the time all the permanent teeth come in at age eleven or twelve. Dental malocclusions (crooked teeth) are the result of the poor facial growth that has been allowed to continue unabated. Some might even call this "supervised neglect!" The most common facial growth problem is underdevelopment of the upper jaw, or maxilla, which leads to crowded teeth, overbites and underbites. These are the most common reasons parents seek the services of an orthodontist in the first place.

Waiting until the patient is near puberty gives the traditional orthodontist more of a challenge than necessary. When facial growth has not been ideal and the bone structure is inadequate to contain all the permanent teeth, the traditional orthodontist believes that to straighten the teeth, as many as four permanent teeth might need to be extracted. They think this because they were taught this in their specialty training. Since the teeth need more bone structure to be in proper alignment, traditional orthodontists mistakenly think that extracting some teeth will create more stability for the remaining teeth after treatment. This is not the case. In fact, this approach might necessitate additional treatment when the patient is an adult. There are other much better options.

Fortunately, this traditional approach is less in favor today than it was more than thirty years ago when I first progressed to my current thinking. I will explain better options than "extraction orthodontics" later. But it's important to understand the traditionalist approach because you are likely to encounter this type of thinking when seeking an orthodontic consultation.

LIMITATIONS OF TRADITIONAL ORTHODONTICS

The following are possible undesirable effects that can occur when permanent teeth are extracted as part of the traditional approach to overcrowding:

1. **Small smiles:** The most obvious effect is that it creates a smaller smile. Even though the fewer teeth left may be straight, the patient still has a narrow upper jaw and a less-than-exceptional smile.

2. **Spaces:** Spaces where teeth were removed can re-open later and cause problems with eating. It can even cause gum disease.

3. **Tongue room:** The space that the tongue occupies will be reduced which can lead to instability of the treatment results and have profound health implications later, even leading to snoring and Obstructive Sleep Apnea.

4. **Nasal obstruction:** Compared to non-extraction treatment, the upper jaw is reduced in size, compounding an already compromised nasal airway and its breathing capacity. This fact can also be a major factor in causing future Obstructive Sleep Apnea.

5. **Recessed jaw:** The lower jaw can be compromised too, making it appear recessed—which is not an attractive look.

6. **TMJ issues:** If not corrected properly, misaligned teeth can lead to TMJ dysfunction, possible later Obstructive Sleep Apnea or snoring issues, and even neck and back problems resulting from head posture compensations. For further information on this, please see *Straight Talk about Crooked Teeth* available at Amazon.com.

7. **Wrinkles:** Extracting teeth can cause a "sunken" look in the lip area. As an adult, this can lead to a wrinkling of the lower face.

The traditional approach, even without extractions, can be detrimental to a child's future.

1. **Difficult corrections:** With a "wait to treat" approach, malocclusions (crooked teeth and jaw structures) are allowed to become more severe before treatment starts, making them harder to correct. The long-term result may be more unstable. Retainers might be needed for the rest of a person's life.

2. **Alignment problems:** With less-than-perfect alignment, the patient's future health and the attractiveness of the smile can be compromised.

3. **Facial imbalances:** Traditional treatment rarely corrects facial structural imbalances, including upper jaw underdevelopment, except by using invasive surgery.

Fortunately, there is a better way:
the future of orthodontics is

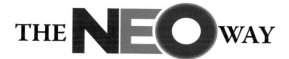

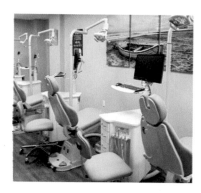

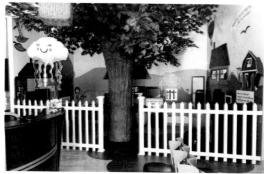

Traditional Orthodontics office   *NEO New Early Orthodontics office*

IT'S DIFFERENT AT NEO

As soon as you enter a NEO office you will recognize that this place is different and has little resemblance to a regular "dental" office. With its colorful, cartoon-type atmosphere, you can tell this is a kid-friendly place. Yes, we provide serious, even life-changing treatment for our patients, but we do our best to make it a fun experience for every child. We want our patients to look forward to their monthly visits with their myofunctional therapist and really get excited to get the results mom and dad are making possible with their financial support.

WHY EMBRACE NEO'S NEW EARLY ORTHODONTIC TREATMENT?

Eighty percent of children will need orthodontics at some point, so there may be only a small chance of avoiding this need. Why take the chance of a child needing much more complex treatment later on?

NEO's philosophy is to start the treatment as soon as the child is old enough to cooperate, which can be as early as age four or five.

In most cases, malocclusions (crooked teeth and jaw structures) are the result of poor oral *myofunctional habits* in the developing child—the way the child uses the muscles in the mouth. It is possible to correct these destructive habits (such as tongue positioning) with proper guidance. This is what we do at NEO: instruct, guide and motivate! The earlier these habits are corrected, the better chance there is of more ideal facial growth.

AGE ARGUMENT FOR NEW EARLY ORTHODONTIC TREATMENT

- At age three, half of facial growth is complete!
- At age seven, 70 percent of facial growth is complete.
- At age twelve, when traditional orthodontic treatment often begins, 90 percent of facial growth is complete.

A question to consider: Instead of waiting until facial growth is almost complete to begin treatment, what if we could have a positive influence on facial growth by starting to correct poor oral habits much earlier? The parent and the orthodontist can work together to help the patient form a better face and teeth alignment early on while there is time to have an influence on facial development.

REASONS FOR MALOCCLUSIONS DEVELOPING

- **Nutrition**: Malocclusions (crooked teeth and jaw structures) have been linked to the changes in nutrition from natural whole foods to refined foods that are now an unavoidable part of the Standard American Diet (SAD). This is certainly one reason so many children have malocclusions these days. What can we do? Good nutrition can be a great start, but there is still more attention needed.

- **Bad habits:** Malocclusions have also been strongly linked to poor oral habits such as mouth breathing and poor tongue habits. Fortunately, changing these poor habits early can significantly improve facial development allowing the teeth to come in straight naturally. This is what we do at NEO!

- **Pressure:** Dr. Melvin Moss, an orthodontist and facial development researcher, proposed the ***Functional Matrix Theory*** about seventy years ago. He wrote that, in dental matters, "form follows function:" a persistent pressure will cause a change in shape of a facial structure over time. This is the essence of why myofunctional therapy works. In addition to using myofunctional therapy training, NEO provides an oral appliance that the child wears while sleeping (when most growth occurs). This combination makes treatment very effective at improving facial growth and correcting facial imbalances.

UNDERDEVELOPMENT OF THE UPPER JAW CAUSES MALOCCLUSIONS

The primary reason for malocclusions occurring in the first place is poor development of the upper jaw. This is the culprit in almost all malocclusions, causing crowded teeth, overbites and underbites. How does this happen?

1. **Tongue posture:** The normal resting position of the tongue is at the roof of the mouth. In growing children, this tongue position stimulates the roof of the mouth to grow. The primary cause of an underdeveloped or narrow upper jaw is a low tongue posture.

2. **Mouth breathing:** When a patient breathes primarily through the mouth instead of the nose, his or her tongue must drop down for the air to pass

over it during breathing. This creates a low tongue posture and a lack of stimulative pressure at the roof of the mouth. This, coupled with the outside pressure of the cheeks pushing inward, causes an imbalance of pressures resulting in narrowing of the upper jaw over time.

3. **Short frenulum:** The tongue is anchored in the mouth by the lingual frenulum, a thin strip of tissue. If the frenulum is too short, the patient might be "tongue tied" which means this strip of tissue will not allow the tongue to rest in its normal position at the roof of the mouth. As we've noted, a low tongue posture can cause a constricted upper jaw. Being "tongue tied" can even make it hard for a baby to breastfeed. I write about this in the book later.

4. **Misuse:** Other poor myofunctional habits, such as thumb or finger sucking and lip biting, can also cause a misshapen upper jaw over time.

MEDICAL BENEFITS OF NEO TREATMENT

The benefits of new early orthodontic treatment go well beyond the teeth and jaw structures. There are many medical conditions, including some not readily apparent, caused or exacerbated by the oral dysfunction that can be improved with NEO's help.

Correctable conditions that have been shown to be related to oral dysfunction include:

- **Sleep disordered breathing:** This category includes every adverse sleep condition from mild snoring to obstructive sleep apnea. These can be serious problems and can lead to other troublesome issues if left unresolved.

- **Mouth breathing:** This habit leads to a reduction of oxygen delivered to the body. Studies have shown that mouth breathers experience as much as a 40 percent reduction in oxygen being exchanged from carbon dioxide in the lungs. The ability to breathe through an unobstructed nasal passageway is vitally important. Without proper nasal breathing, a child's normal growth and development, including the brain, cannot take place. This is especially apparent in a child's facial development, with elongation of the lower face and a gummy smile being the most obvious signs. For a child to reach full mental and physical potential, proper nasal breathing must be established at all costs—period!

- **Hypertrophy of tonsils and adenoids:** If a child breathes mostly through the mouth, the nose cannot filter inborn air properly. This will lead to increased upper-airway infections that will cause swelling of the tonsils and adenoids, compounding the blockage of the airway. Restoration of nasal breathing can help reduce the size of swollen tonsils and adenoids causing their shrinkage over time.

Anatomical Pictures of Facial Structures

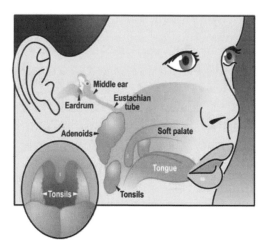

Internal workings of the oral/pharyngeal cavity

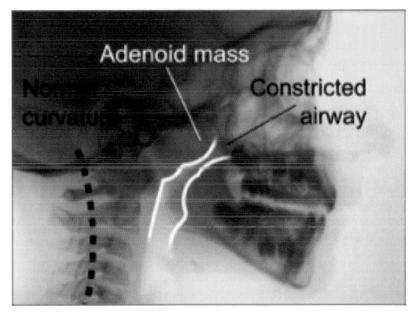

Tonsils or adenoids can block the nasal airway

If the nasal passageways are not clear, resulting in mouth breathing, this condition can result in the following consequences:

- **Chronic sickness:** The nose is designed to catch and filter out many microbes a child encounters. Mouth breathing bypasses this important filter leaving the child exposed to more illness-causing germs.
- **ADD/ADHD:** These psychological and behavioral conditions can be related to mouth breathing and the lowered oxygen levels that result. Many patients have resolved behavioral issues by opening the nasal passageway, resulting in a higher oxygen level in the body.
- **Antisocial behavior:** Like ADD/ADHD conditions, some social problems can be related to improper breathing and low oxygen levels. Mouth breathing can even reduce a child's IQ!
- **Bedwetting:** Bedwetting has been shown to be related to low oxygen levels and can be caused by a mouth-breathing habit. Breaking a mouth-breathing habit has resolved many bedwetting problems.

- **Asthma:** Asthma is a condition that affects breathing. It includes narrowed airways (bronchospasm), a swollen or inflamed respiratory system and abnormal immune system reactions. Opening the upper airway to normal nasal breathing has had a positive effect in resolving asthma.

In addition to mouth breathing and airway dysfunction, a constricted upper jaw can lead to the following:

- **TMJ Dysfunction (TMD):** A narrow upper jaw can result in the "trapping" of the lower jaw causing an overbite and receding lower jaw. This in turn can lead to jaw joints that don't function well (TMJ Dysfunction). More than sixty different adverse health conditions can result from TMJ Dysfunction.
- **Obstructive Sleep Apnea (OSA):** The most common type of sleep apnea, OSA occurs in more than 20 percent of people over age fifty, but it can occur at any age. Sudden infant death syndrome (SIDS) has been linked to OSA.
- **Spinal dysfunction:** When the lower jaw goes back (becomes *retrusive*), as a response, the head will adjust into what is called forward head posture. Over time, this will cause the loss of the natural curve in the neck which can then cause imbalances in the rest of the spine. This is significant. If not corrected, a forward head posture keeps getting worse, ending in a stooped-over condition in old age. This can significantly reduce a person's life expectancy. Please observe the chart below.

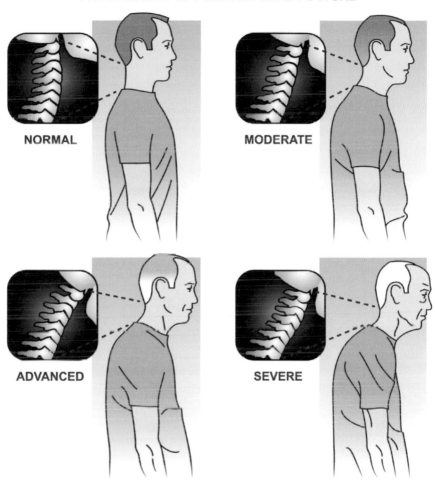

PROGRESSION OF FORWARD HEAD POSTURE

NORMAL

MODERATE

ADVANCED

SEVERE

Note: TMJ, sleep apnea and spinal problems often can be positively influenced by the treatment protocol referenced in this book. These results have either been demonstrated in published clinical studies or are the author's personal observations over the last forty years in clinical practice. For further information, see the author's book *Straight Talk about Crooked Teeth.*

THE NEO NEW EARLY ORTHODONTICS PROGRAM

The Critical Role of the Myofunctional Therapist (MFT)

Throughout this book we will be making references to Myofunctional Therapy. In order to be successful in our treatment, which includes that perfect smile, you will come to understand the critical need to educate both the parent and the child in the proper functioning of the nose, lips, cheeks and tongue. Fun exercises to teach habits of proper breathing, swallowing, tongue and lip posture, and even head posture, are taught. This specialized educator role is filled by a highly trained Myofunctional Therapist, a most critical position at NEO. You will see a number of references for this work throughout the book.

NEO Protocol for Evaluation and Treatment at Any Age

Birth to Age Three: What Should a Parent Look For?

Although we do not begin NEO appliance therapy at this early age, many parents find it valuable to begin thinking about their newborn child's oral habits. NEO educates parents to make sure the stage is set for ideal growth and development. What should a parent look for?

Nasal breathing is healthy breathing

You need to make sure the baby breathes silently with his or her mouth closed. Any obstruction must be cleared as soon as possible so nasal breathing can be reestablished. If not corrected, mouth breathing results in less oxygen to the brain and other body parts. This can be very dangerous for the developing baby, as neurological growth at this stage is occurring rapidly. Ninety percent of neurologic growth is completed by age five. This type of growth precedes facial and body growth (sixty percent facial growth is reached by age five).

Mouth breathing causes many problems

Mouth breathing is perhaps the most devastating of the preventable problems a newborn can have. Parents should make it a number-one priority to ensure their baby has unrestricted nasal breathing. They should remain vigilant as the child grows to make sure proper nasal breathing continues.

An upper-airway restriction may develop due to the following causes:

- Enlarged tonsils and/or adenoids caused by airway infections which can block the upper airway;
- Enlarged adenoids may block the Eustachian tube leading to middle ear infections.
- Allergies may cause constricted airways and
- After several years of poor facial growth, an underdeveloped upper jaw can make mouth breathing worse.

Whatever the cause, the nasal obstruction must be eliminated so that normal nasal breathing is established.

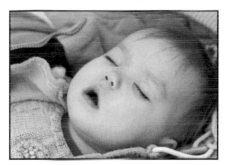 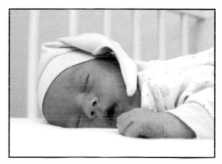

Pictures illustrate babies heading for trouble because of mouth breathing

Breastfeeding is highly encouraged

Breastfeeding is much better for the baby nutritionally and is highly recommended for at least the first six months, and even up to two years after birth, for several important reasons:

- Confirmed in studies, breastfeeding also provides a host of systemic health benefits from helping to prevent childhood lymphoma and leukemia to increasing cognitive development and disease immunity.
- According to the World Health Organization, if all newborn babies were breastfed within one hour of birth, given only breast milk for their first six months of life, and continued breastfeeding up to age two, the lives of approximately 220,000 children would be saved per year.

Breastfeeding also results in better oral and facial development

When the baby nurses, oral muscles are exercised. Strong facial muscles help to promote more ideal facial growth and development. This happens because in the suckling process the baby needs to push the nipple up against the roof of the mouth with his or her tongue to expel the milk from the breast. This is the ideal posture of the tongue that promotes normal upper jaw growth, helping to prevent crooked teeth, overbites and underbites.

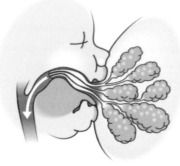

These pictures show a proper latch with negative pressure to express milk, the tongue pressing the nipple against the palate and proper tongue extension over the jaw bone.

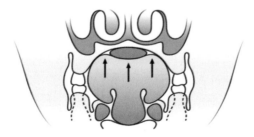

Sometimes breastfeeding is not possible. A common reason for baby's inability to breastfeed may be that the tongue is attached to the lower jaw by a short frenulum, a condition we have described as "tongue tied" and which is formally known as akyloglossia. A dental professional can quickly evaluate this condition by sweeping a finger under the tongue to see if there is a problem.

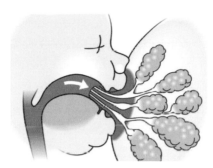

Tongue tie can make breastfeeding unpleasant, but can also
lead to underdevelopment of the upper jaw, producing malocclusions

Tongue tie exists in 5-10 percent of the population, yet some patients are never treated for this condition which continues into adult life. Common symptoms for older patients include the following:

- Cannot extend tongue straight out of the mouth, but tongue curves down
- Cannot raise tongue to roof of mouth
- Difficulty in swallowing, grimacing present
- Speech problems

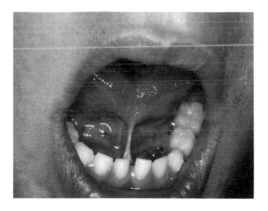

Tongue tie example in a young child

- If a tongue tie is present, it can be easily treated by a procedure called a frenectomy. A dentist or orthodontist can perform this relatively simple surgical procedure. Newer laser correction of tongue ties are quick and comfortable for the child. If you suspect your child has this condition, we can evaluate it and solve the issue for him or her.

- An untreated tongue tie can have a significant negative affect on a child's facial growth by preventing the child's tongue from resting in a healthy position at the roof of the month. This in turn changes the structure of the upper jaw. Significant tongue ties must be corrected as early as possible, ideally soon after birth. We use state-of-the-art science laser techniques at NEO to make this correction as comfortable as possible for the child, helping to ensure the stability of future orthodontic treatment.

Bottle-feeding can produce malocclusions

Studies have shown that there is a strong correlation between exclusive bottle-feeding and the development of malocclusions. This may be due to the following:

- The baby's nutrition may be sacrificed. Earlier we wrote about the effect of the Standard American Diet (SAD) on the development of malocclusions.

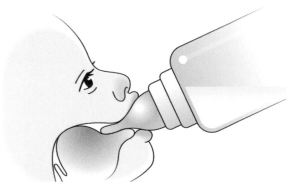

- When a baby bottle-feeds, the bottle may have excessive milk flow causing the baby to thrust his or her tongue to push out the bottle when satisfied. This can cause the development of an adverse swallow pattern and a tongue-thrust habit which are primary causes of malocclusions.

- The size of the nipple may be obstructive and can prevent the normal tongue posture that is so important in the proper development of the upper jaw. Note the picture below.

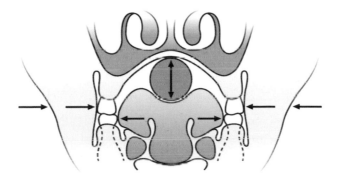

Bottle feeding causes the tongue to be in a lower posture
and may cause a tongue thrust habit

Ages Four to Ten: Getting Started, Going the Distance

Decision Time: Upper Jaw Expansion or NEO's Nighttime Myofunctional Appliance (NMA)

If extreme upper jaw constriction exists when the child comes for treatment at this age, the jaw may need to be expanded before treatment with NEO's positioning appliance. The expansion can also be performed later if needed. Your orthodontic professional will help you decide.

NMA Treatment

NEO's actual treatment can begin with the NMA, assuming the patient and parent are ready to comply with the habit-correcting activities we show them. Wearing the appliance for one hour during the day, plus while sleeping at night, gives us the best results in correcting all adverse myofunctional habits.

Getting Started

1. The treatment plan emphasizes the correction of adverse oral habits to facilitate ideal facial growth. The child, under the guidance of the Myofunctional Therapist (MFT), learns activities to create positive habits with breathing, tongue function, lip seal and so on.

2. The NMA should be worn one hour while awake plus through the night.

3. Monthly appointments keep the plan on track. The Myofunctional Therapist (MFT) sees the child once a month for a two-year period. Under the direction of the doctor, the MFT eventually replaces a softer NMA with a more rigid one. The patient may have as many as three to four appliances during the two-year period of the prescribed treatment time. This program has proven very effective with millions of children.

NEO utilizes a system well-proven around the world

- At NEO New Early Orthodontics we use a system for early treatment that is now being used by dentists in more than 100 countries with millions of children receiving the benefit.
- We at NEO are now spreading the good word about this revolutionary treatment.

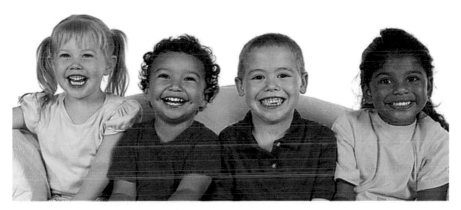

Most children show signs of incorrect dental and facial development at an early age. Two of these children have a mouth-breathing habit and two have an incorrect swallow pattern. They are great candidates for NEO's New Early Orthodontics program.

The NEO Way begins with seeing the patient at a young age when most facial growth is still ahead. This evaluation might begin with observations by the parent or consultations with the physician. A NEO dentist can even evaluate a newborn baby.

As stated before, Dr. Melvin Moss's Functional Matrix Theory—now universally accepted by orthodontists throughout the world—states that where teeth are concerned, "form follows function." Any persistent pressure will change the facial structure over time. This is the essence of why wearing the NEO appliance while sleeping, along with myofunctional therapy exercises, is so effective.

A BETTER WAY!

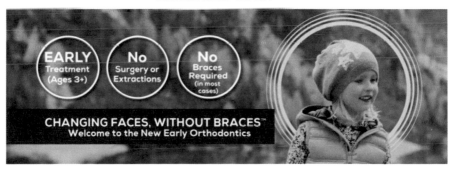

Mom, I don't really want braces!

NEO New Early Orthodontic treatment works naturally with a child's growth

- **Night treatments:** Most growth occurs while the child sleeps so NEO treatment can be most effective very early with a nighttime appliance.
- **Early growth:** Somatic (facial) growth is rapid during the child's early years when physiologic structural changes can be greatly influenced.
- **Habit changes:** Learning is easier for the child at this age. Life is less complex and parents are more in control. Bad habits are not yet ingrained, so they can be eliminated. The earlier treatment begins, the easier it is to establish positive habits.
- **Keeping it fun!** NEO myofunctional therapists make sure the learning activities are always fun for the child so that he is excited to come to his monthly visits.

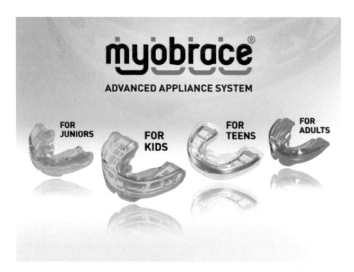

NEO'S NIGHTTIME MYOFUNCTIONAL APPLIANCE (NMA)

NEO uses the Myobrace, an appliance now gaining worldwide recognition, as its nighttime appliance. It is best for not only teaching children new, healthy oral habits, but also for shielding the inward pressures of the cheeks to allow much better growth of the dental arches. When we refer to NEO's Nighttime Myofunctional Appliance (NMA), we are talking about the use of the Myobrace.

The pediatric Myofunctional Orthodontic evaluation

We recommend that all children have a myofunctional evaluation by age four. An orthodontist—or pediatric orthodontic dentist and myofunctional therapist (MFT)—can complete a thorough examination to determine whether the lower facial structures are functioning properly.

The evaluation includes:

- **Proper nasal breathing:** Is breathing silent? If the parent hears the child snoring or choking, a breathing disorder is present and must be evaluated to determine the cause. This is a serious problem at an early age because it can get much worse as a child develops.
- **Tonsils and adenoids:** These structures are evaluated for size and to determine if they are obstructive to nasal breathing. Establishing nasal breathing can help shrink the tonsils and adenoids, possibly eliminating the need for surgical removal.
- **Tongue posture while swallowing and resting:** Is the tongue pushing between the teeth when the patient swallows? Is swallowing difficult for the child?
- **Lip posture:** Are the child's lips closed while resting and sleeping? If not, mouth breathing is occurring. Does the child close the lips while swallowing? Does swallowing cause a grimace? If so, this indicates mentalis muscle hyperactivity and an adverse swallowing pattern.
- **Head and body posture:** Does the head remain in a forward thrust position? This can be an indication of overbites and mouth breathing.
- **Jaws and teeth:** Does the child have a constricted maxilla (upper jaw)? Is a deep bite, open bite or crossbite observable?
- **Adverse habits:** Does the child suck on thumbs or fingers, bite fingernails or chew on pencils?

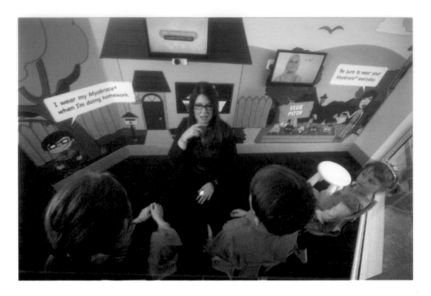

The MFT works with the patient during monthly visits to coach and encourage the child to participate in treatment every day. The MFT gives "homework" for the child and parent to do daily using apps. The MFT also requests doctor checks every three to four months, or as needed when changing to a new appliance.

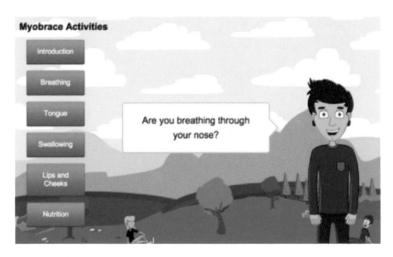

NMA Myobrace activities have strong interactive programs which parents can put on their smart phones to help kids with their "homework." The exercises take only a few minutes a day. Consistency is the key.

NEO KIDS CLUB MEMBERSHIP CARD

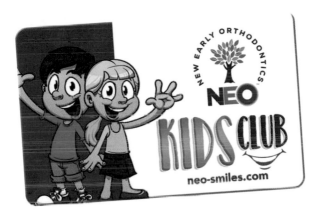

NEO Kids Club: We use rewards to help encourage cooperation. Our young patients are excited to be a part of NEO Kid's Club where they can work to gain rewards and have other fun benefits such as supervised parties. NEO is a celebration of a better life.

FUN PRIZES TO WIN WITH NEO KID'S CLUB

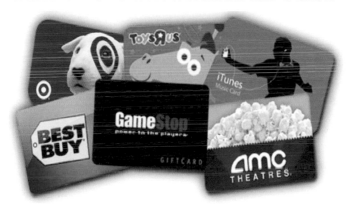

Patients accumulate points from successful appointments at NEO— whether at the office or with video conferencing. They can use their points to buy prizes from cooperating vendors. We are not above bribing children to get their cooperation if a healthy, beautiful smile is the result. We call that a Win/Win for all! It is The NEO Way!

Going the Distance

What happens when the initial treatment period is over? After the child has finished our twenty-four-month program, we monitor the dental development carefully.

- **Recall visits:** We like to schedule a visit every four to twelve months until all permanent teeth come in. During this time, the patient is encouraged to continue wearing the nighttime Myobrace and practicing the corrected habits learned during the initial program.

- **Is it time for braces?** When all permanent teeth have erupted— except the third molars, known as "wisdom teeth"—we evaluate the child to decide if further treatment is indicated. Of course, the patient and family always have the final say, but this is the right time to do any finish work to get the best possible result. Most patients who successfully complete the twenty-four-month NMA protocol do not need braces. But sometimes, wearing braces for even a brief period of several months can be enough to make the smile perfect. If we see unusual dental development, such as impacted teeth, missing teeth or extra teeth, we can suggest more comprehensive treatment to address these issues.

Long-term stability is a major advantage with NEO. Our patients are less likely to need to wear retainers for the following reasons:

1. **Bad habits resolved!** By participating in regularly scheduled myofunctional office visits, a child is able to eliminate adverse habits that cause malocclusions to develop in the first place.

2. **Good facial development:** The facial structures form more ideally, allowing permanent teeth to come into the mouth in better alignment. This creates better long term stability.

3. **Less relapse:** Therefore, less braces correction means less dental relapse, since alignment is better from the start.

The NEO approach also has other advantages:

1. **Keep the teeth!** It eliminates the need to extract permanent teeth by helping the patient develop a more ideal dental arch.

2. **Forget the surgery.** It eliminates surgeries to correct improperly grown facial structures.

3. **Enjoy natural balance.** It creates better facial balance in a more natural way.

Ages Eleven, Twelve and Beyond: Alternatives and Additional Treatment

At this stage of a child's development, 90 percent of facial growth has occurred. Their final, permanent teeth are now coming in. This is when many traditional orthodontists are just beginning their treatment.

As stated before, for those families doing it the NEO Way, this is the time to assess whether braces will be needed to finish treatment or if nothing more is indicated. Most successful Myobrace patients will not need further help with braces, but if they do, the time they will need to wear braces should be greatly reduced. The decision for use of additional treatment with braces always rests with the parent and patient.

Most treatment plans will include the option of finishing with braces at a reduced fee. The combination of myofunctional treatment plus braces, in most cases, does not exceed the normal cost of braces alone.

When an alternative to the Myobrace is needed

If the patient comes in for treatment after most growth is completed, it might be desirable to use what is called Functional Facial Orthopedics to correct facial and dental structures instead of NMA treatment. Treatment of this type will generally be needed when starting in the teen years and may be followed by braces or Clear Aligner treatment. Conditions such as missing or extra teeth or impacted teeth can make the Myobrace difficult or impossible to effectively use. It is still very important to make sure any adverse habits are corrected to ensure future stability. The patient might need myofunctional therapy, with or without a NMA appliance, during a braces phase of treatment.

We'll share some examples of this later treatment option in the case studies in Part II B. In all cases, the doctor's evaluations will determine the proper treatment for the child.

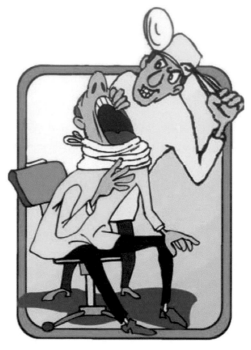

"Orthodontics does not have to be as painful as pulling teeth."

An additional note regarding treatment with the Myobrace System

It has been said by many practitioners throughout the world that as much as 80 percent of children treated with the Myobrace will not need further orthodontic treatment (braces) when the final permanent teeth come in. This is truly terrific news for many children because it means they can avoid the traditional braces route.

Although this may be true for many parts of the world where function and health are the main concern, in the United States, the desire for the perfect straightness of the teeth may set a different standard. If this is the case, then the 80 percent rule might not be realistic—but 50 to 60 percent probably is. In other words, more than half the children who receive early treatment in the US will not need further orthodontics.

At NEO, the patient is followed with routine visits until all primary teeth have been lost and the last permanent teeth (except wisdom teeth) come into the mouth. This usually happens at age eleven or twelve when the bicuspids and the twelve-year molars are expected to come in. An evaluation by the orthodontic doctor will reveal one of three possibilities:

Three scenarios for the future:

1. **Perfection!**

   If all teeth have come in straight and with proper function, then no further treatment is needed and stability will be outstanding.

2. **Almost perfect.**

   Teeth might have come in well, but minor tweaking can make the mouth more perfect. In this case, in consultation with the doctor, the parent and patient might decide to either leave well enough alone, or they might feel a few months of braces would be worthwhile to enhance the result. The parent/patient always has that choice. If they decide that some time in braces is worthwhile, then additional fees would apply.

3. **A little way to go.**

   Because of the complexity of the case or a lack of patient cooperation, a more comprehensive approach is indicated. A separate fee for this would apply. Our NEO commitment to our patients is this: If the patient has cooperated with treatment at least 80 percent during the NMA phase of treatment, our fee for additional orthodontics (credited with the initial NMA phase fee) will not exceed what the average fees would be for a more traditional, full orthodontics approach. As stated before, this won't apply to cases where missing, extra, or impacted teeth are present.

This arrangement is a great benefit to the parents of a child. There is nothing to lose here. NEO does this because we know that, with proper NMA wear and compliance with exercises, the difficulty of the orthodontic treatment will be significantly reduced. That means less time and cost for the NEO office AND for the parents—another Win/Win situation. This is The NEO WAY!

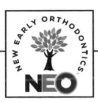

PART II A
NEO New Early Orthodontics Case Studies

CASE 1

FOUR-YEAR-OLD GIRL WITH OPEN BITE, CROSSBITE, TONGUE THRUST

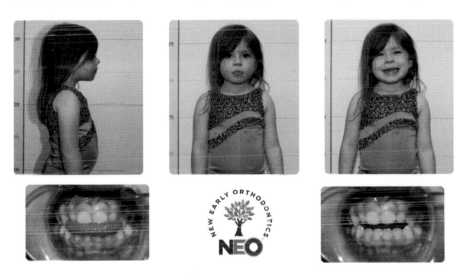

Before NEO treatment

This four-year-old child had a major problem with poor tongue posture, creating a significant open bite and a lower jaw that positioned itself to her left. These problems can only get worse if ignored. The upper jaw was developing smaller than normal, creating what is known as a "crossbite."

Through proper myofunctional exercises, aided by a Myobrace appliance (worn while sleeping plus one hour in the evening), this beautiful young lady was able to create better oral habits. NEO solved the problem in less than a year. Please see progress photo next page.

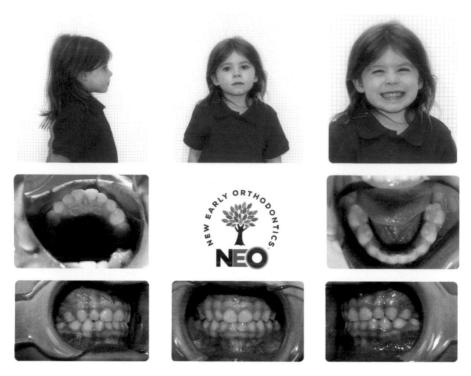

After ten months of NEO treatment

Normal development is now possible because, once the patient established ideal orofacial habits, growth will work in our favor. The anterior open bite is now closed and the posterior crossbite is corrected. We do still have work to do correcting the small jaws to create room for larger permanent teeth to come in, but thankfully, we have a number of years ahead before this will become an issue.

CASE 2
SEVEN-YEAR-OLD BOY WITH OVERBITE AND LOWER CROWDING

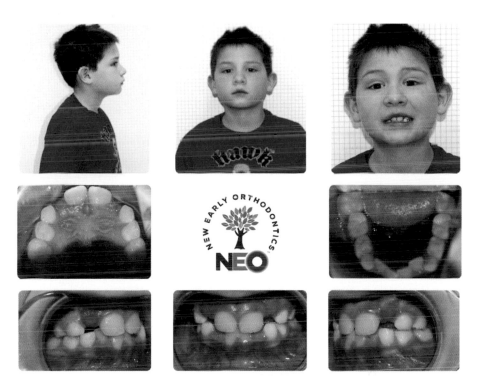

Before NEO Treatment

This seven-year-old boy had a mouth-breathing habit and his resulting low tongue posture caused a lack of support for his developing upper jaw. This had caused a narrowing of the upper jaw resulting in an overbite and lower crowding. Compensating muscle overactivity and an incorrect swallowing pattern were noted. Other health related issues included headaches, speech impairment, and behavioral and social delays.

NEO treatment included activities with our MFT to correct the adverse habits. The patient responded well to our treatment which included one hour plus nighttime Myobrace wear. The following photo series was taken six months after the beginning of treatment.

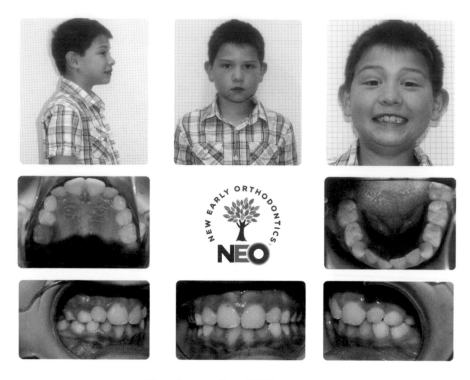

After six months of NEO treatment

Note the great improvement of overbite and dental crowding. After six months, myofunctional habits had improved and the child's head posture and lip competence were more normal. His social skills even got better during treatment! When improvement takes place in a relatively short time, both the patient and parent are motivated to continue.

CASE 3
SEVEN-YEAR-OLD GIRL WITH LARGE OVERBITE

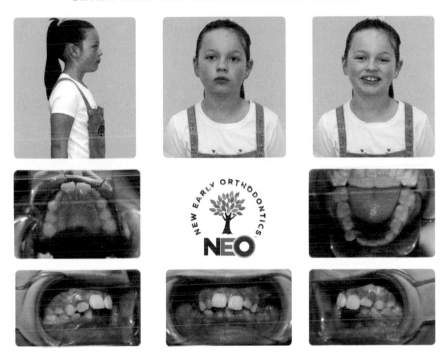

Before NEO treatment

This seven-year old girl had a very significant overbite. She was a mouth breather which caused low tongue posture and contributed to a recessed lower jaw. She also had severe constriction in the upper arch with night time clenching and grinding. In addition, we discovered she had a lateral tongue thrust, incorrect swallowing pattern and poor lip posture. Previous health concerns revealed a history of ear infections and gastrointestinal issues.

Six months of excellent patient cooperation produced such an outstanding result, it surprised even us.

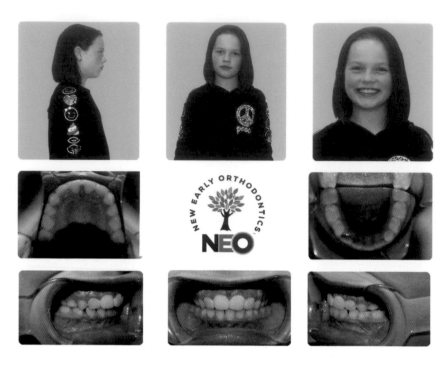

After six months of treatment

The excellent result here speaks for itself. A great patient always makes us look good! This patient may avoid braces in the future.

CASE 4

EIGHT-YEAR-OLD GIRL WITH DENTAL CROWDING AND POOR MYOFUNCTIONAL HABITS

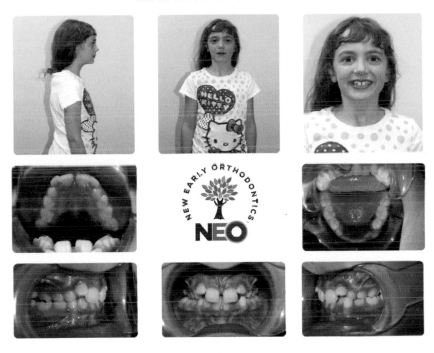

Before NEO Treatment

Our eight-year-old patient began NEO New Early Orthodontics treatment with the following conditions: Severely constricted upper jaw, forward head posture, and harmful myofunctional habits including thumb sucking, mouth breathing and reverse swallow. After finishing a two-year program with monthly myofunctional therapy sessions, aided by overnight and one-hour daily wear of a Myobrace, she attained the result shown in the following photos.

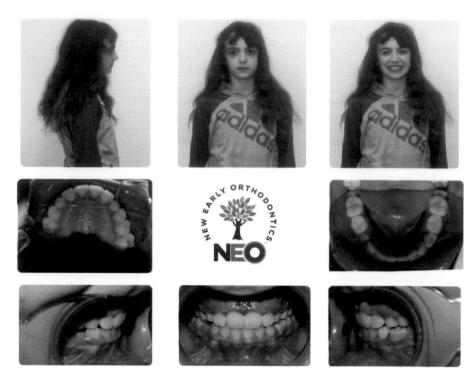

After twenty-eight months of NEO treatment

This composite series of photos, taken twenty-eight months after beginning treatment, shows a patient who likely will not need any traditional braces. Because the adverse myofunctional habits had all been corrected during treatment, her remaining teeth will have room to come in straight. Her dental stability will be outstanding for the rest of her life with no retainers needed. This child will always be grateful to her parents for the early investment they made in her future smile and health.

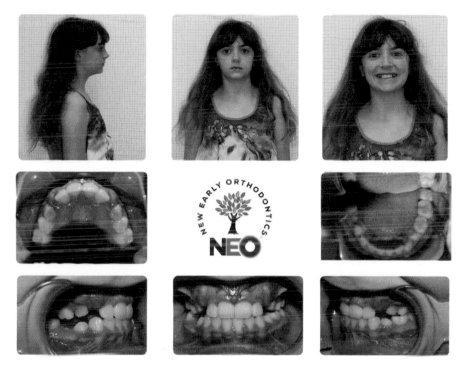

After thirty-five months of NEO treatment

Our NEO New Early Orthodontics treatment protocol is a twenty-four-month program. We continue to follow each patient after this period of time until all teeth have come into the mouth in order to determine the need for possible additional work with braces. Since this patient lives in Michigan with her family, most of her appointments were handled by video conferencing. This is a very common practice in our office; we see many out-of-state patients from the West to East coasts and everywhere in between.

From a practical standpoint, we typically will see the patient at the evaluation appointment and at office visits for appliance changes every four to six months. We have found this system to work very well and our long-distance patients appreciate the early treatment expertise we have at NEO.

CASE 5

NINE-YEAR-OLD GIRL WITH EXTREME CROWDING AND OVERBITE

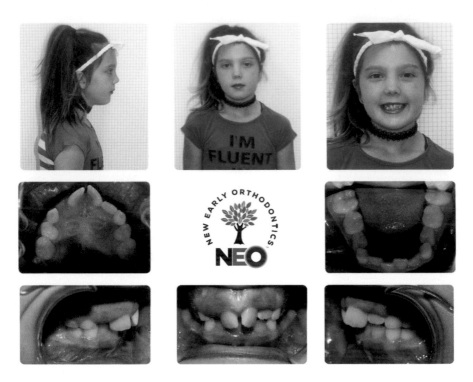

Before Treatment at NEO

This nine-year-old girl began NEO New Early Orthodontic treatment with severely constricted dental arches and a large overbite. Her jaw joints (TMJ) were out of alignment which caused significant clicking, and she had a "tongue tie" (excess lingual frenum) that restricted the tongue's normal resting position at the roof of her mouth. She had a forward head posture and exhibited myofunctional dysfunction that included mouth breathing and anterior tongue thrust with an adverse swallowing pattern. She also had allergic "shiners" implying airborne allergies were a factor. The following composite photos were taken after thirteen months of myofunctional therapy with nighttime myobrace wear.

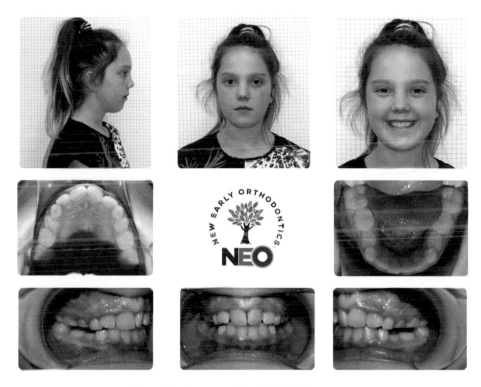

After thirteen months of NEO Treatment

When these photos were taken, the patient had completed thirteen months of treatment with a Myobrace appliance and myofunctional therapy. Significant improvement was already apparent, including much better arch forms and elimination of TMJ clicking and mouth breathing. She showed some improvement in head posture, although more will occur in the future.

CASE 6
NINE-YEAR-OLD BOY WITH THUMB-SUCKING HABIT

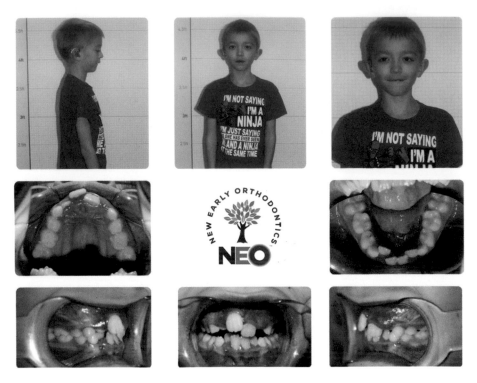

Before NEO Treatment

This nine-year-old boy began treatment with a thumb-sucking habit and many other adverse myofunctional habits including incorrect swallowing pattern with anterior tongue thrust and mouth breathing. He had a high palate with significant upper and lower arch constriction and lower dental crowding. He had developed an open bite by sucking his right thumb. This dysfunctional pattern was creating significant neuromuscular pain and headaches.

Our treatment with the Myobrace, and myofunctional therapy for twenty months, made significant improvement in both form and function, as evidenced by the following composite photos of his mouth.

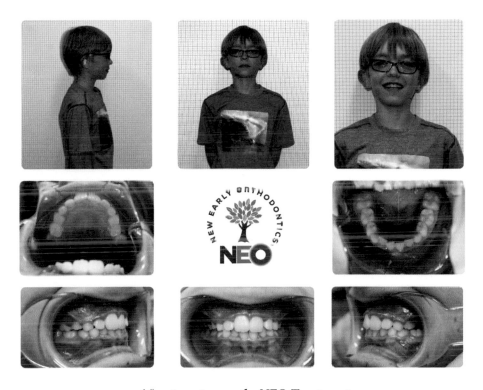

After twenty months NEO Treatment

Note the broadened upper and lower arch forms and the improvement in dental crowding. The headaches are now gone and he functions better overall.

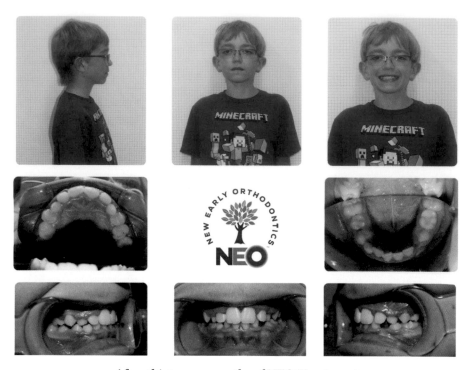

After thirty-one months of NEO Treatment

This patient might never need braces. What a mess was avoided by not waiting to treat! If you go back and look at the pictures from before treatment, you can see that we are well on our way to avoiding braces!

CASE 7
NINE-YEAR-OLD BOY WITH DEEP OVERBITE

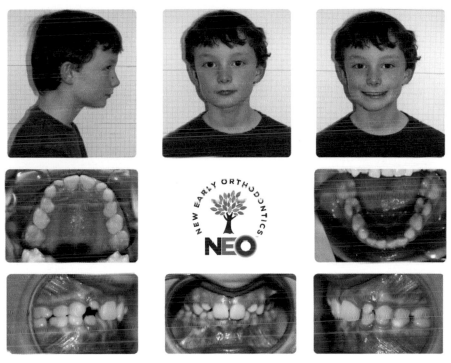

Before Treatment at NEO

This nine-year-old boy had a history of clenching, grinding and nail biting before beginning treatment with the Myobrace appliance. These adverse habits were working against a favorable growth pattern and typically would mean at least a few years of braces to "fix" the damage. NEO had a better way!

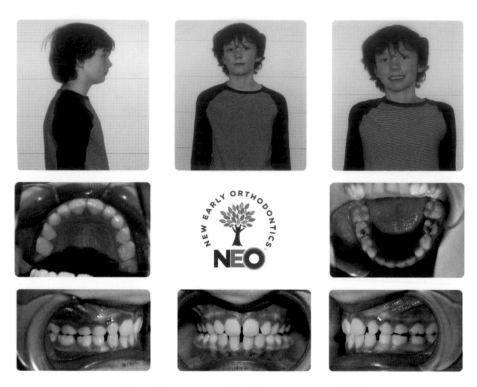

After thirteen months of treatment at NEO

This is a progress photo taken after thirteen months of treatment with nighttime Myobrace wear. Note the increased fullness of the dental arches which are now expanded and have adequate room for the new permanent teeth to come in. His overbite is now reduced to normal and all adverse myofunctional habits have been eliminated. This young boy might avoid braces when the remaining teeth come into his mouth.

CASE 8
TWELVE-YEAR-OLD GIRL WITH EXTREME 11MM OVERJET

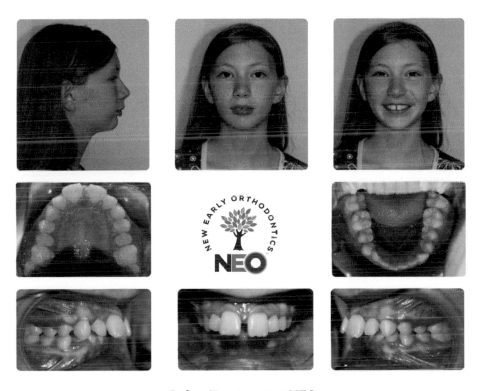

Before Treatment at NEO

This twelve-year-old patient had an anterior tongue thrust and an extreme overbite (11mm). Her parents were told by several orthodontic specialists that she would need surgery—which would have been the traditional approach. The patient was highly motivated to improve her facial appearance and avoid surgery. NEO had a better way!

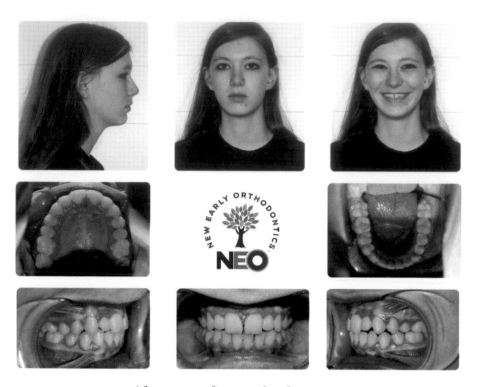

After twenty-five months of treatment

The patient wore a simple, removeable jaw expander for six months, and then the Myobrace at night plus one hour of daytime wear for the duration of her treatment. Notice how the patient's arch form has been broadened and her extreme overbite has been completely corrected.

Braces were an option in this case, but the patient wanted a perfect result, so she wore braces for the next seven months. She finished with an ideal result—and no surgery was ever needed!

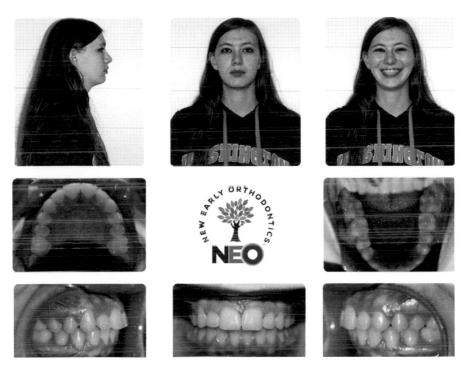

After seven months of braces (following twenty-five months of Myobrace)

A note to help understand this revolutionary treatment:

The cases shown are typical of the dramatic changes that can occur with this early treatment method. However, we want to make very clear that these marked changes are only possible with very good patient compliance. Without good patient compliance, the results will not be what you see here and the opportunity to really make a difference can be lost. For that reason, working with a highly trained myofunctional therapist—like the ones at NEO—is a critical element in the education and motivation of the patient.

Please also understand that the Myobrace appliance, although very important, is not the primary driver of NEO New Early Orthodontic treatment success. The main factor in successful treatment is patient compliance and family support in doing the necessary myofunctional exercises as directed by the NEO myofunctional therapist. Myobrace is used to help treatment be more effective. After all, in most cases, problems with alignment of the teeth and jaws developed because of adverse oral habits such as poor tongue positioning. The patient must un-learn these habits and learn new, positive oral habits to allow the mouth to develop properly.

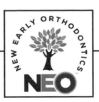

PART II B
The Lauson System
Cases Ages Thirteen to Eighteen

Depending on a patient's age, treatment with a nighttime-only appliance like the Myobrace can be challenging. The Functional Facial Orthopedics (FFO) techniques of The Lauson System can now take over to help the patient achieve a great result. The following cases were all treated by Dr. Lauson and are included in his book *Straight Talk about Crooked Teeth*. Note the following cases:

CASE 9
THIRTEEN-YEAR-OLD MOUTH BREATHER WITH CROWDED MOUTH

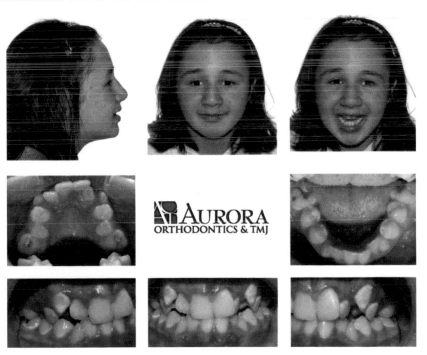

Before Treatment

This patient began seeing us at age thirteen. She was a chronic mouth breather which had caused her upper jaw to be substantially underdeveloped and constricted. As stated before, for a mouth breather, the habitual resting tongue posture is lower than the ideal posture. A patient breathing properly through the nose rests the tongue high against the roof of the mouth so the inhaled air can't pass over it. A mouth breather's low tongue position creates a neuromuscular imbalance: the forces of the cheek muscles that push inward override the outward pressures of the tongue causing constricted development of the upper jaw. This can cause crowding of the patient's teeth. It bears repeating: the underdeveloped maxilla (upper jaw) is the root cause of almost all malocclusions (crooked teeth, overbites and underbites).

A traditional orthodontic approach would likely have included the removal of the patient's four bicuspid teeth. Then the remaining teeth would have been straightened even though it would be impossible to achieve a broad, beautiful smile. Although the teeth would be straight, there would be four fewer teeth. The constriction of the upper jaw and the nasal airway challenges would remain.

This treatment type, which we can call "extraction orthodontics," also has long-term negative consequences; an increased susceptibility to TMJ dysfunction, an increased likelihood of obstructive sleep apnea, and even future neck and back problems. We avoided all these potential negative consequences for this patient in this way:

1. Our patient was treated with Functional Facial Orthopedic (FFO) expansion appliances—called upper and lower Schwarz appliances—which use slow palatal expansion (SPE) over a period of nine months. The Schwarz appliance is a removable acrylic appliance that is activated once every three days. This is not to be confused with rapid palatal expansion (RPE) in which an appliance is typically fixed to teeth and activated (enlarged) daily. Rapid palatal expansion has been shown to be unstable and is not recommended. For further information on this, please refer to *Straight Talk about Crooked Teeth* available through Amazon.com.

2. We used straight wire braces for the next sixteen months to give the ideal result shown below.

3. All treatment objectives were accomplished including the elimination of the mouth-breathing habit and lowered tongue posture. No permanent teeth were removed.

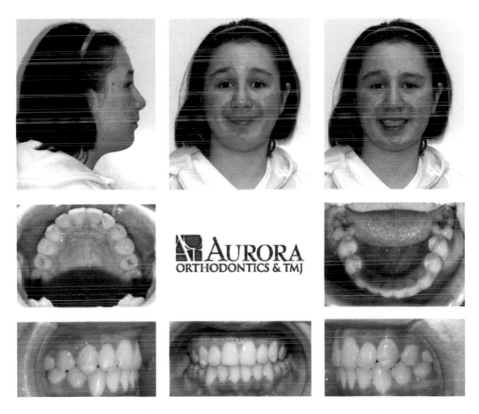

After twenty-five months of treatment with the Lauson System

CASE 10
FOURTEEN-YEAR-OLD GIRL WITH EXTREME CROWDING

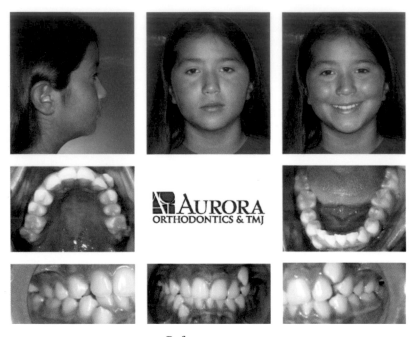

Before treatment

A narrow, underdeveloped upper jaw had prevented this fourteen-year-old patient's permanent canine teeth from coming in. Please see the panoramic X-ray below. She also had a TMJ click on her right side, a signal of a dysfunctional jaw joint (TMJ).

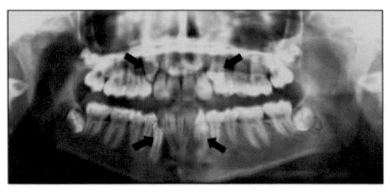

Pretreatment panoramic x-ray showing blocked-out cuspid teeth

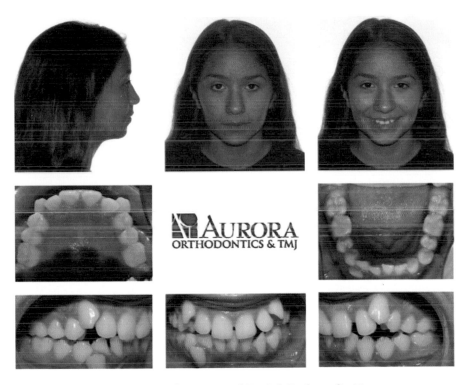

After nine months of Functional Facial Orthopedic Treatment

Nine months of her treatment had created a good deal of bone structure enhancement, but we needed to gain even more space to straighten the teeth with braces. After this phase, braces were placed for fifteen months. Many practitioners do not realize the value of FFO treatment and therefore would likely have removed four permanent teeth in order to straighten the remaining ones. This would have left narrow arch forms, and the treatment might have contributed to future TMJ pain and other problems.

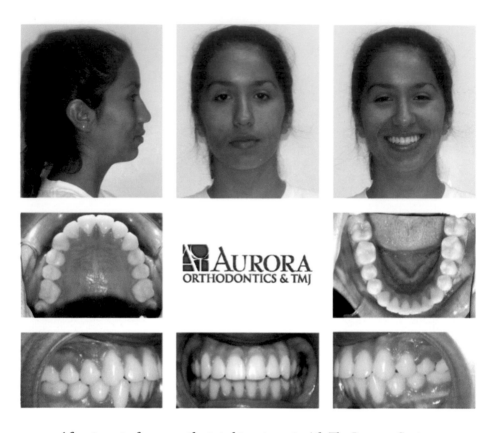

After twenty-four months total treatment with The Lauson System

*Note: Many dental professionals do not take the clicking jaw joint seriously. Unfortunately, because of a lack of training given in dental schools, unless a dentist has taken further TMJ training, he or she won't be able to adequately address the problem of TMJ dysfunction.

CASE 11

TWELVE-YEAR-OLD WITH UNDERBITE GIVEN ONLY SURGERY OPTIONS

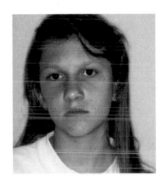

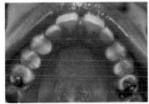

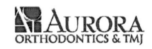

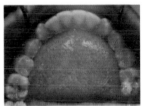

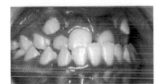

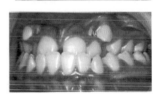

Before treatment photos

Surgery is not always the best or only option

This patient had a dilemma. The orthodontists she consulted had agreed she should wait until about age sixteen, when her facial growth was complete, to have surgery that would entail "breaking" her lower jaw so it could be moved back to its proper position. She would then be fitted with braces. This was not an appealing idea to either the parent or the child. Then the family stumbled upon an article I had written for a local community newspaper that explained the "magic" of FFO. The article explained that many skeletal problems, where a deficiency of bone structure exists, can be corrected without surgery using the techniques we are discussing here.

The mother and child agreed to our treatment and we proceeded to treat her over the next two years. The initial FFO phase was performed using a maxillary three-way sagittal appliance. The purpose of this FFO appliance was to not only widen the deficient upper jaw, but also to bring the premaxilla more forward to correct its deficiency and provide bone structure to correct the anterior crossbite. This was accomplished over the next nine months at which time braces were placed. The final braces portion took another fifteen months resulting in a total treatment time of twenty-four months.

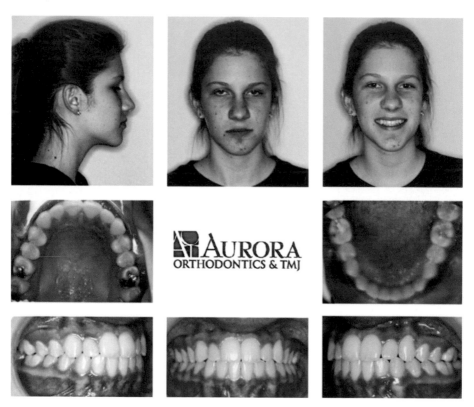

After twenty-four months of treatment at completion

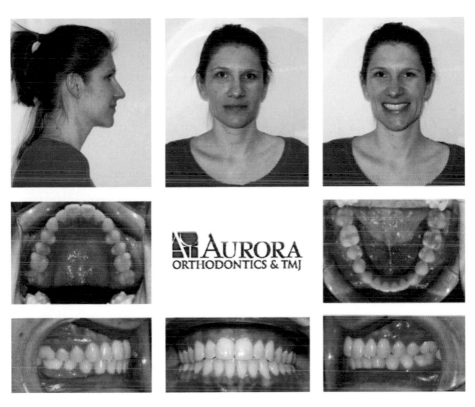

Photos taken at age thirty-four

Photos taken seventeen years after completion of orthodontic treatment. This patient's smile has improved with age!

Note: A much more extensive list of completed cases is shown in the book by Dr. Lauson, *Straight Talk about Crooked Teeth*, which is available through Amazon.com. The primary purpose of *The Neo Way* is to educate the parents of young children, making them aware of NEO New Early Orthodontics. We created this book to show parents the truly revolutionary way orthodontics can help their children to have a better life in the future. These last three cases demonstrate our ability to get great results even with the older patients. However, older patients require much more effort and expense to get these results. We encourage parents to treat their children early, both to save money and achieve lasting, natural results.

Why not treat orthodontic problems in the most natural way possible? See you at NEO!

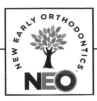

PART III
The Lauson System:
Ten Keys to Facial Harmony

At NEO, we use *The Lauson System: Ten Keys to Facial Harmony* as the objective. We do our best to create each of the ten keys for each patient. Many of the cases shown in the previous pages were much more difficult to treat than the average. We included them to demonstrate that it is possible to achieve outstanding results even in difficult cases.

As we pointed out before, good patient cooperation is critical. Without it, the great results shown would be impossible to achieve. But these techniques are special. Even with excellent patient cooperation, the treatments used in more traditional orthodontics would not provide these results.

The Lauson System is based on ten keys to facial harmony, essential goals in achieving maximum benefit to the patient, not only from an aesthetic standpoint, but also in creating total body health. The satisfying part of using this system is that it can produce "movie star" smiles while avoiding surgery or extraction of permanent teeth.

Straight Talk about Crooked Teeth, by Dr. Kent Lauson (published in 2012 and available through Amazon) is a book about possibilities that take orthodontics to a new level. When the keys to facial harmony are reached, the results can be life-changing. The book is replete with endorsements from prominent doctors and testimonials from patients who now have the smiles they always wanted. It also explores how that same system has successfully treated TMJ dysfunctions while having a positive impact on other medical conditions such as ADHD, asthma and obstructive sleep apnea.

As confirmed by thousands of successfully treated cases over more than thirty years, Functional Facial Orthopedics (FFO), combined with braces or clear aligners, can solve almost all dental occlusion and lower facial harmony problems—without subjecting the patient to surgery or removal of any permanent teeth. Since the original book was published, I have seen the need to add an additional key and have revised the order of the original nine keys. Key #3: Treat as Early as Possible, was added to address my long standing concern about letting malocclusions develop unabated if there was effective treatment that could be started much earlier than traditional treatment timing. This is where the Myobrace system shines because it allows appliance treatment to begin as early as age four. Knowing that we have this early option for treatment allows us to assess patients much sooner, ensuring that even newborn babies can have a better chance to develop properly.

When reviewing the 10 Keys, understand that there is some overlapping of objectives since lack of one key can precipitate other developmental problems and can compromise one or more other keys. Another way of saying this is: The accomplishment of one key, such as Proper Nasal Breathing, makes it easier to accomplish other keys like Healthy TMJ Function or Ideal Head Posture.

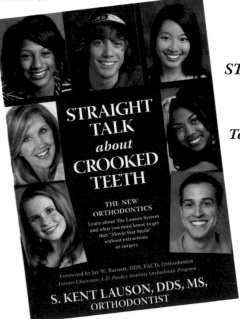

STRAIGHT TALK ABOUT CROOKED TEETH
The Lauson System:
Ten Keys to Facial Harmony

KEY #1: UNOBSTRUCTED NASAL BREATHING

Unobstructed nasal breathing is the number-one key because a person's quality of life is so dependent on it. Proper breathing is paramount in having normal facial development and it's also vital to so many other areas of health considerations. It is almost impossible to overemphasize its importance. Breathing obstructions, for whatever reason, must be evaluated and eliminated. Obstructed nasal breathing can lead to mouth breathing which can then lead to many unnecessary problems including poor facial and dental development. The primary causes of nasopharyngeal obstruction are allergic rhinitis (allergies), deviated septum, underdeveloped upper jaw and obstructive tonsils or adenoids.

KEY #2: CORRECT ADVERSE ORAL MYOFUNCTIONAL HABITS

As many as three out of four children have adverse oral myofunctional habits. These bad habits include anything that places abnormal pressures within the oral cavity because pressure can influence facial growth in a negative way. The most common of these habits is mouth breathing which causes the tongue to rest low in the mouth. The tongue should rest against the roof of the mouth where it stimulates normal upper jaw growth. The underdeveloped upper jaw is almost always responsible for bite and alignment problems that require orthodontics. Other oral habits that are destructive include improper swallowing, poor tongue or lip posture, thumb and finger sucking, lip biting, and chewing on objects like pens, pencils, or even ice.

KEY #3: TREAT AS EARLY AS POSSIBLE

Eighty percent of children will need orthodontics at some point in their lives. NEO's philosophy is to treat as early as patient cooperation can be established. As we have explained, malocclusions needing correction are mainly the result of poor oral myofunctional habits. Poor nutrition also can be a factor, but since there is abundant available information regarding nutrition, our focus is to inform the parent about the effects of poor oral myofunctional habits. With proper guidance, bad habits can be corrected allowing for more ideal facial development. The earlier these habits are corrected, the better the result. This concept is well explained earlier in this book.

KEY #4: FULLY DEVELOPED UPPER JAW (MAXILLA)

The upper jaw holds the key, in many ways, to facial beauty as well as the proper function of the lower face and teeth. The upper jaw should be wide and full to accommodate all fourteen normal upper teeth (excluding wisdom teeth) in proper alignment and to provide proper lip support. The patient's full smile should not show a lot of gum tissue or expose dark triangles between the teeth and the cheeks. The maxilla can be expanded with slow palatal expansion (SPE) at any age as the cranial sutures—including the mid-palatal suture—remain flexible throughout life.

The following case is a good example of the use of FFO to expand the maxilla to an ideal shape to create a handsome, movie star smile. This patient was sixteen years old when treatment began. He had substantial crowding of his front teeth. His upper jaw was narrower than what is considered ideal. Traditional orthodontics typically would have recommended the removal of four bicuspid teeth and then straightening of the remaining teeth with braces. The recommendation might also have been made to use maxillofacial surgery to achieve the desired result.

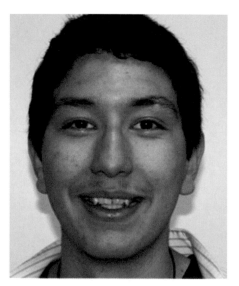
Pre-treatment facial photo

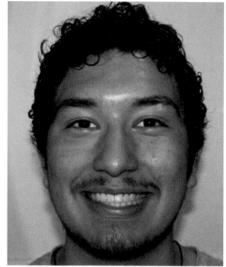
Post-treatment facial photo

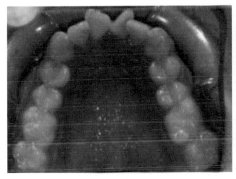 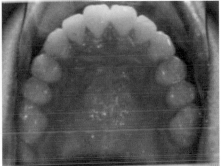

Pre-treatment roof of mouth   *Post-treatment roof of mouth*

Instead, Functional Facial Orthopedics helped expand his palate to make room for all his teeth. After treatment was completed, the patient's smile was full and confident. This result would not have been possible without the expansion of the arch forms.

KEY #5: PROPER POSITIONING OF LOWER JAW (MANDIBLE)

The lower jaw should be in balance with the upper jaw. The most common imbalance happens when a narrow upper jaw forces the lower jaw back, trapping it in a recessed position. This is called "retrusion" and can cause an undesirable overbite and overjet. This malocclusion can lead to TMJ dysfunctions, forward head posture, or even obstructive sleep apnea. With lower facial balance, teeth can be positioned ideally and facial harmony can be established.

KEY #6: HEALTHY TMJ FUNCTION

The TMJ, or temporomandibular joint, is the joint on each side of the face in front of the ear. These joints allow us to open and close the jaws so we can speak and eat. The TMJ is the most complex joint in the human body.

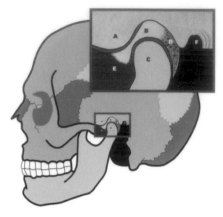 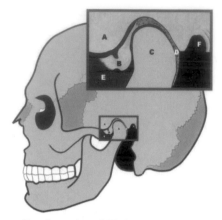

Normal anatomy of TMJ   *Dysfunctional TMJ anatomy*

The TMJs can become dysfunctional if they are strained by the positions of the teeth which can force the lower jaw out of alignment and into a pathologic position. The TMJs are the cornerstone of a proper bite and if they are dysfunctional they must be corrected. If not, a myriad of symptoms—including headaches, facial pain, clicking jaw joints and problems with the eyes and ears—will appear and worsen over time. To establish a healthy balance for the chewing system, function of the TMJ must be taken into consideration.

KEY #7: IDEAL HEAD POSTURE

As we discussed earlier in this book, proper head posture has an important impact on neck and back health as we discussed earlier in this book. Teeth and jaw positions profoundly influence head posture. If proper balance is achieved with the first six keys above, then head posture can be positively influenced. As an additional benefit, further care from a neck and back doctor or therapist also can be more effective.

KEY #8: AVOIDANCE OF OBSTRUCTIVE SLEEP APNEA

Obstructive Sleep Apnea (OSA) is a serious medical problem affecting as much as 20 percent of the population. It is now unrefuted that OSA can lead to heart disease and premature death due to strokes, heart attacks, or choking in the night. Recent studies have even shown links between OSA and cancer and Alzheimer's Disease. In OSA, restricted airflow during sleep can cause a person to stop breathing causing an apnea event, which can happen hundreds of times per night. The most common reason for OSA is when the lower jaw is recessed too far back, although a narrow upper jaw also might be involved. By properly following the keys listed, the possibility of OSA can be reduced in severity or avoided altogether.

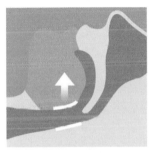 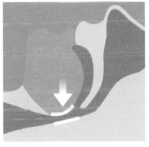 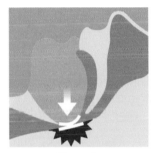

Normal   Snoring   Obstructive Sleep Apnea

KEY #9: IDEAL LOWER FACIAL SYMMETRY

Facial asymmetries can develop because of a mismatch of the upper and lower jaws and dental malocclusions which can cause the lower jaw to shift to one side or the other. A narrow upper jaw is almost always the source of this type of asymmetry. A correction should be made early in life to prevent complications such as a TMJ dysfunction from developing later on. The chapter on this important key shows how easy it is to misdiagnose this problem which can result in unnecessary surgeries used to correct an asymmetry.

KEY #10: OPTIMAL TEETH POSITIONING

Crowding or spacing of front teeth is the most obvious malocclusion that an untrained eye can easily see. However, for the trained orthodontist or dentist, problems with how the jaws come together must be addressed. Crossbites, overbites and underbites are less obvious, but can impact health. Decades ago, Dr. Larry Andrew's *6 Keys to Normal Occlusion* established a guideline for dental specialists to use regarding this topic, assuming the full complement of twenty-eight teeth is maintained and that permanent teeth are not extracted during orthodontic treatment.

The Lauson System: Ten Keys to Facial Harmony was developed over the last forty years in private practice. By following the goals in this system, it is my belief that the patient can achieve the healthiest, most beautiful and most stable results—without having to endure permanent teeth extractions and surgery. Whenever possible, all ten keys are treatment goals for every patient.

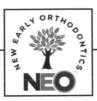

Dr. Kent Lauson's Story

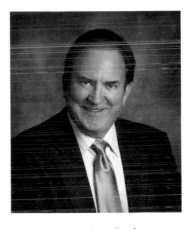

Dr. Lauson is a traditionally trained specialist in orthodontics who came into the field because he wanted to straighten teeth and create beautiful smiles. The first years after specialty training, he practiced in Denver, Colorado and performed orthodontics. Initially, he performed treatments like most of his colleagues using primarily braces. Many of his patients needed extractions to straighten their teeth. However, after a few years in practice, he became aware of unexplained problems some of his previously treated patients were experiencing. Those problems included headaches, facial pain and jaw joint pain. He wondered, "Could this have anything to do with what I did to straighten the teeth?" This was very upsetting to him because he not only didn't know the answer to this question, but he also was unaware of how to help these patients. More questions came up and he was motivated to find the answers.

He began a five-year journey (averaging eighteen trips per year) traveling to professional seminars to find much-needed answers. He went to not only dental and orthodontic seminars, but also to allied medical meetings in the fields of otolaryngology, physical therapy, chiropractic, massage therapy and even craniosacral therapy. He knew there was a connection between the various fields and he began finding many of the answers he sought. Things would never be the same as he now realized that treatments he had been doing for patients were in many ways responsible for the negative side effects they were later experiencing.

Since becoming enlightened, Dr. Lauson has successfully treated thousands of patients who were dealing with significant challenges. He discovered how to effectively treat these problems, and if they occurred as part of orthodontic treatment, how to get them corrected during the treatment. Unfortunately, this information is not part of current orthodontic education, so these problems remain widespread even today.

Several realizations have come to Dr. Lauson during this time:

- Traditional orthodontic training, which he and most other orthodontists originally received, concentrates primarily on "straightening the teeth" and does not seriously recognize that dental health and treatment can have a profound effect on the rest of the body.
- Braces can effectively straighten teeth, but they cannot significantly change bone structure that is either deficient or out of alignment. For this, special types of functional facial orthopedics can be valuable. Special devices can solve many skeletal problems without surgery.
- It is much easier, more cost effective, and more stable long term to prevent malocclusions (crooked teeth, overbites, and so on) from developing in the first place rather than to "wait to treat" until all the permanent teeth have come in, as many traditional orthodontists do.
- By doing early evaluations on children from age three to make sure only positive oral habits are established, it is possible to stop malocclusion development in its tracks. New Early Orthodontics (NEO) treatment can begin as early as age four with emphasis placed on ideal oral myofunction. Treatment includes ideal habit training and a series of monthly sessions with a therapist.
- This treatment is not yet well-known in the United States. NEO plans to expand the development of clinics for NEO New Early Orthodontics® brand throughout the United States and Canada.

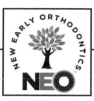

NEO New Early Orthodontics
contact information:

www.NEO-Smiles.com 303-690-0400
www.NewEarlyOrthodontics.com 303-690-0100

COMPLIMENTRY COPIES OF *THE NEO WAY*!

A complimentary copy of THE NEO WAY is available to any patient of NEO New Early Orthodontics. Just check in at your office for your copy.

Non-patients of NEO may receive a complimentary digital e-book version of The NEO Way by sending an email to:

info@NewEarlyOrthodontics.com

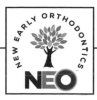

Praise for Dr. Lauson's previous book, *Straight Talk about Crooked Teeth*, from prominent orthodontists and dental specialists

"Timely and insightful, this profound work is brilliant in its simplicity. Dr. Lauson cuts to the core, outlining the real connection between the human airway, mouth breathing, crooked teeth, TMJ disorders and latent disease. *Straight Talk about Crooked Teeth* clearly outlines how to achieve the coveted movie star smile with a deeper understanding of how debilitating conditions like obstructive sleep apnea, ADD/ADHD, bedwetting and headaches can be avoided. It is refreshing to finally have these important lessons and concepts in one easy-to-understand book for every parent, patient, dentist and physician who really cares about straight teeth, healthy TMJs, quality of life and longevity. Colleagues, it is time for my beloved dental profession to not only change lives with a winning smile, but more importantly, to SAVE LIVES!"

J. Brian Allman, DDS, Noted author and lecturer, Diplomate, American Board of Dental Sleep Medicine, American Academy of Pain Management, Director, TMJ Therapy and Sleep Center of Nevada, Reno, NV

"The book *Straight Talk about Crooked Teeth* should be mandatory reading for every orthodontic provider in the United States and Canada. This book should also be read by every parent contemplating making an orthodontic investment in his or her child's future health and well-being. Its principles embody the fundamentals of what is necessary for long-lasting, highly cosmetic, and highly functioning results which, if not followed, will result in only a compromised solution to the presenting orthodontic problems. I can only pray that Dr. Lauson's treatment principles will seep deeply into the conscience of the world's orthodontic profession."

Brendan C. Stack, DDS, MS, Orthodontist, noted author and lecturer Vienna, VA

"I have personally had a very similar understanding and conclusion regarding the current state of orthodontics. The concepts so clearly presented can help patients avoid unnecessary extractions of permanent teeth and jaw surgery. I commend Dr. Lauson for his efforts to advance orthodontics in a more functional and stable manner than traditional orthodontics allows. To think more and do things differently than the conventional wisdom, teachings and methods say marks true progress. We can provide superior results for our patients by evaluating each of them as a whole system, a complete person, not just their teeth. It is my hope that this book and Dr. Lauson's thinking become the mainstream in orthodontics; then orthodontics will have a great impact to improve the attitude, self-esteem and overall health of people everywhere. I highly recommend *Straight Talk about Crooked Teeth!*"

Lloyd Truax, DDS, MSD, Orthodontist, author, and lecturer
Founder and 1st Chairman, Mayo Clinic Orthodontic Department
Rochester, MN

"Dr. Kent Lauson's book, *Straight Talk about Crooked Teeth*, is an excellent resource for parents, patients, doctors and dentists. Dr. Lauson clearly explains the connection between a beautiful smile and the keys to overall health. Dr. Lauson is a university-trained specialist in orthodontics and has spent his career building on this education and finding synergy from related medical and dental fields in order to more effectively help his patients. Now these years of study, work, and real-world application are set forth in an easy-to-understand guide. When followed, the principles that Dr. Lauson describes will not only result in maximum facial aesthetics, but also the best foundation for lifelong optimal health. I have spent my career helping people who suffer with TMJ problems, facial pain and sleep apnea. I applaud Dr. Lauson for publishing information that I know will help many people avoid such problems and help parents make informed decisions that will help their children avoid such problems later in life."

Jamison R. Spencer, DMD, MS, Noted lecturer and author
of Small Airway, Big Problem: How Sleep Apnea
Often Goes Undiagnosed in Women, Children, and Skinny Dudes
President, American Academy of Craniofacial Pain, Diplomate, American
Board of Craniofacial Pain and American Board of Dental Sleep Medicine
Boise, ID

"Dr. Lauson has done an excellent job of integrating the orthodontic-TMD-sleep connection in the treatment of his patients. This book clearly illustrates why orthodontic clinicians must embrace the functional, nonextraction philosophy. Failure to deal effectively with TMD and sleep apnea with our orthodontic patients can result in serious health problems in the future. I would encourage all clinicians who want to diagnose and treat holistically to read this book. Dr. Lauson shows many successfully treated patients throughout the book. It is a must read for patients as well as all orthodontic clinicians who want to improve the quality of their patients' lives."

Brock Rondeau, DDS, Noted author and lecturer of orthodontics,
TMJ dysfunctions, and dental sleep medicine
President, Rondeau Seminars
Ontario, Canada

"It is nice to finally see an orthodontic text written in patient-friendly language that comprehensively looks at the entire craniofacial complex and not just the fit of the teeth. For dental professionals and patients alike who are interested in the intimate relationship between teeth, jaw joints, muscles, airway and posture, this book is a must read. Clearly and concisely put together, Dr. Lauson has made a strong case for the use of functional facial orthopedic techniques and the 'nine keys' to not simply create a prettier smile, but to have long-lasting, positive effects on the overall health of the individual in ways not often associated with dental treatment. *Straight Talk about Crooked Teeth* will be prominently displayed in our reception and consultation areas as an invaluable piece of patient education."

Dan Demmings, DDS
British Columbia, Canada

"I would recommend this book for any parent contemplating orthodontic treatment for his or her child or any adult who is unsure which brace option is the best for him or her. This book dispels some of the myths associated with 'traditional orthodontics,' such as 'don't treat till the child has all his or her adult teeth' or 'extractions of premolar teeth to resolve crowding is the ideal treatment solution.' This book is long overdue as it also links the medical/dental interface, e.g., nasal airway obstruction, TMD, snoring/OSA, and maligned jaws. Dr. Lauson must be applauded for his continual search for answers beyond the confines of his traditional training. His results speak for themselves."

Derek Mahony, DDS, MS, Orthodontist, author,
and international lecturer
Sydney, Australia

"Spot on! This is the book every mother should read before choosing an orthodontist for her family. Most practitioners doing orthodontics don't pay enough attention to the airway and TMJ. The nine keys to lower facial harmony should be part of every graduate orthodontic curriculum. Why not have a more beautiful smile while opening the airway, alleviating headaches and clicking jaws, and improving posture. A must read for every parent, dentist and orthodontist."

Michael Gelb, DDS, MS
Clinical Professor, NYU College of Dentistry
New York City, NY

"Dr. Lauson has completed a timely and wonderful book for the orthodontic patient, as well as for the orthodontic practitioner. His many years of experience have enabled him to develop a system for optimal orthodontic treatment. A full smile that retains all permanent teeth and creates an optimum airway is the enviable goal for orthodontic professionals and their patients. *Straight Talk about Crooked Teeth* is a must-read book."

Ron Cook, DDS, MSD, Orthodontist
Educator, Next Generation Orthodontic Education
Lake Havasu, AZ

"This easy-to-read book, specifically aimed at the layperson interested in learning more about options for orthodontic treatment, is written with simple explanations of orthodontic and scientific terms that keep the reader engaged. It presents relevant, reliable information that will help patients and parents choose the best orthodontic options through informed decision making. Dr. Lauson challenges some outdated concepts, using orthodontic literature to support his assertions. The information is presented in a balanced, well-thought-out manner which most fair-minded people will find easy to accept. I highly recommend Dr. Lauson's book *Straight Talk about Crooked Teeth* to anyone who is contemplating orthodontic treatment."

G. David Singh, DDSc, PhD, BDS, Lecturer and author
of Epigenetic Orthodontics in Adults
Director, Smile Foundation, Beaverton, OR

"In all my years in dentistry, I have never seen a book like this; certainly nothing out there is comparable at this time. This book is a "possibility" book—showing that beautiful life changes are possible as a result of the treatment that Dr. Lauson has to share. He has shown that even the most complicated of cases are treatable with predictability when the principles in the book are implemented. I would recommend this book to anyone."

Jay W. Barnett, DDS, FACD, Orthodontist, noted author, and lecturer
Former Chairman, L.D. Pankey Institute Orthodontic Program
Key Biscayne, FL

"Dr. Kent Lauson's book *Straight Talk about Crooked Teeth* hits the nail on the head. As a functionally trained TMJ dentist who has instructed thousands of dentists worldwide, I wholeheartedly agree with the powerful concepts put forth in this book. The Lauson System is clearly explained, and if it's treatment objectives are followed, it will not only allow the creation of beautiful smiles, but will enable treated individuals to live much more healthy and happy lives."

William B. Williams, DMD, MAGD, MICCMO, Lecturer and consultant
Founder, Solstice Dental Advisors
Atlanta, GA

"I give this book two big thumbs up! A well-written and concise guide for people considering orthodontic treatment for their children or themselves; this book not only teaches, it also engages you to read more and understand that there are better ways to accomplish results holistically than traditional methods allow. Dr. Lauson has taken a complex set of ideas and techniques to develop a system that is easy to follow and has excellent results. The multiple aspects of total health as they relate to orthodontics are truly inspiring and are vital information for everyone. The cases presented show the evidence-based results as well as the quality, compassion, and commitment he gives his patients and the years he has spent refining his craft. In my thirty years of working in the orthodontic industry, I have seen many changes and learned a great deal. This book has given me new energy and proves that the envelope is ever expanding; I'm enthusiastic to share this with others. Dr. Lauson is an advocate with an important mission; keep it up."

Kevin Truax
President, Tru-Tain Orthodontics
Rochester, MN

"Dr. Lauson has produced a timely book that was written for parents and patients which helps them to understand the relationship between the head, neck, and in particular the mouth, as it relates to the general health of the individual. He is a professional who has incorporated this holistic approach into his orthodontic practice as it relates to health in general."

David T. Grove, DMD, MS, MSEd, MSc, Orthodontist
Associate Professor of Orthodontics, Next Generation
Orthodontic Education
Las Vegas, NV